HORMONAL AND ALKALINE DIET FOR WOMEN

Reverse Disease and Heal the Body Naturally

Inspired By
Barbara O'Neill

By
Barnabas Noah

Contents

INTRODUCTION

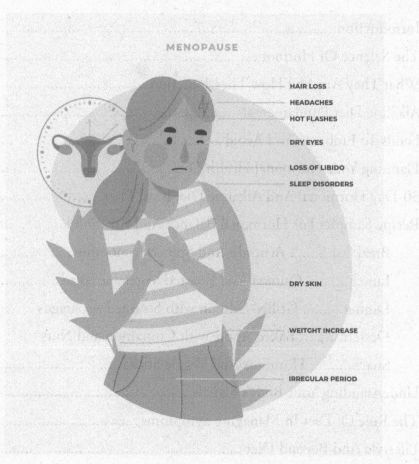

MENOPAUSE

HAIR LOSS
HEADACHES
HOT FLASHES
DRY EYES

LOSS OF LIBIDO
SLEEP DISORDERS

DRY SKIN

WEITGHT INCREASE

IRREGULAR PERIOD

Welcome to "Hormonal and Alkaline Diet for Women," a journey into understanding the profound connection between our diet and hormonal health. In this book, we delve into the world where food is more than just sustenance; it's a key to unlocking the secrets of hormonal balance and overall well-being.

Hormones are like the body's messengers, communicating and orchestrating a symphony of biological processes. From mood regulation to reproductive health, hormones play a pivotal role. However, in the hustle of modern life, hormonal imbalances have become all too common, often leading to a myriad of health issues that affect millions of women worldwide. The good news? The power to positively influence our hormonal health lies significantly within our diet.

This is where the concept of an alkaline diet enters the scene. Imagine your body as a garden. Just as the soil's pH needs to be just right for plants to thrive, our bodies require a balanced pH for optimal health. The alkaline diet, rich in fruits, vegetables, nuts, and seeds, aims to maintain this delicate balance. It's not just about eating healthy; it's about creating an environment where hormones can function at their best.

The benefits of an alkaline diet extend beyond hormonal health. It's associated with increased energy levels, improved digestion, and a stronger immune system. By reducing the intake of acid-forming foods and increasing alkaline foods, we can help our bodies maintain a state of equilibrium, which is essential for overall health and well-being.

Throughout this book, we'll explore the complex relationship between what we eat and how our hormones behave. We'll uncover the secrets of the alkaline diet, provide practical tips for implementing it, and share stories of transformation and triumph. Our goal is to empower you with knowledge and inspire you to take control of your health, one meal at a time.

So, join us on this enlightening journey. Whether you're struggling with hormonal imbalances, seeking to improve your overall health, or simply curious about the impact of diet on your well-being, this book is your guide to a healthier, more balanced you. Let's embark on this path together, towards a life where harmony between diet and hormones is not just a dream, but a reality.

Chapter 1

THE SCIENCE OF HORMONES

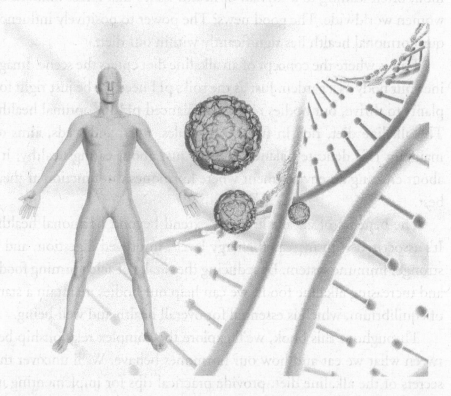

Embarking on a journey to understand hormones feels like unlocking a complex, yet fascinating world within our own bodies. Hormones, those tiny yet mighty messengers, are essentially chemicals produced by various glands in our bodies. They travel through our bloodstream, whispering instructions to tissues and organs, orchestrating a myriad of bodily functions.

Imagine hormones as the conductors of an orchestra, each playing a crucial role in creating harmony in our body's symphony. From regulating our mood, growth, and metabolism to even our reproductive processes, hormones are the unsung heroes in the narrative of our health.

Now, what's truly intriguing is how these hormones interact with what we eat. Picture your diet as a set of keys. Some foods can turn on the engine of certain hormones, revving them up, while others might act as brakes, slowing them down. This intricate dance between our diet and hormones is where the magic, or sometimes the chaos, begins.

For instance, let's talk about insulin, a hormone famous for its role in managing our blood sugar levels. When we consume foods high in sugar, our body releases insulin in response. It's like a traffic cop, directing glucose – the sugar in our blood – to either be used as energy or stored away. But here's the catch: consistently high levels of sugar intake can lead to what's known as insulin resistance, a condition where our cells start ignoring insulin's instructions. This can set the stage for a cascade of health issues.

Then there's cortisol, often dubbed the 'stress hormone'. While it's essential in managing how our bodies use carbohydrates, fats, and proteins, excessive stress can lead to elevated cortisol levels. This can disrupt our metabolism, and sleep patterns, and even lead to weight gain, particularly around the midsection.

It's not just about individual hormones, though. The harmony of our hormonal symphony depends on the balance of various hormones. This balance can be delicate, easily tipped by factors like stress, lack of sleep, and, crucially, our diet.

Understanding this, it becomes clear why an alkaline diet, rich in fruits, vegetables, nuts, and seeds, can be a game-changer. Such a diet can help maintain an optimal pH level in our body, creating a conducive environment for hormonal balance. It's not about radical dietary overhauls, but rather, making mindful, gradual shifts toward foods that nourish and support our hormonal health.

In essence, the science of hormones is a testament to the intricate and beautiful ways our bodies operate. It underscores the profound impact of our dietary choices on our hormonal health, urging us to be attentive to what we consume. After all, in the grand orchestra of our body, maintaining hormonal harmony isn't just desirable – it's essential for a symphony of good health.

Hormones 101

WHAT THEY ARE AND

HOW THEY FUNCTION

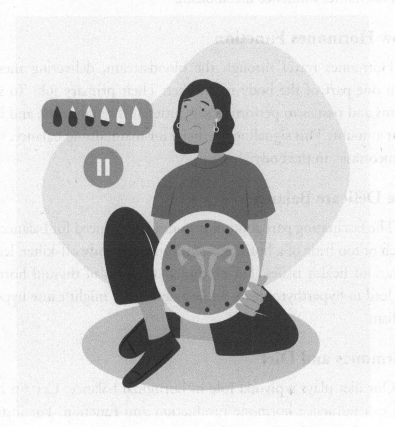

Hormones, those tiny yet mighty messengers in our body, play a role akin to a symphony conductor, orchestrating various bodily functions with remarkable precision. Imagine them as invisible threads weaving through our body, connecting different organs and systems, ensuring everything works in harmony.

The Nature of Hormones

At their core, hormones are chemical substances produced by glands in the endocrine system, like the thyroid, pancreas, and adrenal glands. Each gland has its own set of hormones, tailored like a key to a lock for specific cells and organs throughout the body. For instance, insulin from the pancreas helps regulate blood sugar levels, while thyroid hormones influence metabolism.

How Hormones Function

Hormones travel through the bloodstream, delivering messages from one part of the body to another. Their primary job? To signal organs and tissues to perform their duties at the right time and in the right amount. This signaling is crucial for maintaining balance, or homeostasis, in the body.

The Delicate Balance

The fascinating part about hormones is their need for balance. Too much or too little of a hormone can throw the body off-kilter, leading to various health issues. For example, an excess of thyroid hormone can lead to hyperthyroidism, while a deficiency might cause hypothyroidism.

Hormones and Diet

Our diet plays a pivotal role in hormonal balance. Certain nutrients can influence hormone production and function. For instance, omega-3 fatty acids, found in fish, have been shown to regulate cortisol levels, a hormone linked to stress. Similarly, foods rich in phytoestrogens, like soy, can mimic estrogen in the body, potentially impacting hormonal health.

The Feedback Loop

Another key aspect is the feedback loop system. It's like a thermostat in your house. When hormone levels in the blood reach a certain point, the endocrine glands adjust production accordingly, either ramping up or dialing back. This loop ensures that hormone levels stay within a healthy range.

Hormones and Emotions

Not to be overlooked is the connection between hormones and emotions. Hormones like serotonin and dopamine, often dubbed as 'happy hormones,' have a profound impact on our mood and feelings of well-being. They remind us that hormonal health is not just physical but deeply intertwined with our mental and emotional state.

In summary, hormones are the unsung heroes in our body, quietly yet powerfully steering our health and well-being. They remind us of the intricate interconnectedness within our bodies and the importance of a balanced lifestyle and diet to maintain optimal health. By understanding hormones better, we're not just unlocking secrets to physical health but also paving the way to holistic well-being.

THE IMPACT OF DIET ON
HORMONAL HEALTH

Hormones, the body's chemical messengers, play a pivotal role in regulating various bodily functions. They're like the conductors of an orchestra, orchestrating everything from growth and metabolism to mood and reproductive health. And guess what plays a significant role in this complex symphony? Your diet.

1. Nutrients and Hormonal Balance:

- Proteins: They're not just for building muscles. Proteins are crucial in the production of hormones. Foods rich in protein, like fish, lean meat, and legumes, provide amino acids essential for hormone synthesis.

- Fats: We often demonize fat, but healthy fats are vital for hormonal health. Fatty acids, especially Omega-3s found in fish and flaxseeds, are important for producing hormones and reducing inflammation.

- Carbohydrates: Carbs impact insulin, a key hormone that regulates blood sugar levels. Complex carbs from whole grains, fruits, and vegetables help maintain steady insulin levels, avoiding spikes and crashes.

2. The Gut-Hormone Connection:

- Your gut is a hormonal hotspot. A healthy gut flora aids in the regulation of hormones like insulin, ghrelin (the hunger hormone), and leptin (the satiety hormone). Fermented foods and dietary fiber support gut health, thus influencing hormonal balance.

3. The Impact of Sugar and Processed Foods:

- Excess sugar and processed foods can wreak havoc on hormones. They can cause insulin resistance, leading to a cascade of hormonal imbalances, impacting everything from your mood to your metabolism.

4. The Role of Phytonutrients:

- Certain plant-based foods contain phytonutrients that can mimic or influence hormones. For example, soy contains phytoestrogens that can have estrogen-like effects on the body, beneficial in menopause.

5. Hydration and Hormonal Health:

- Water is crucial for every cellular function, including hormone production and release. Dehydration can disrupt hormonal balance, affecting stress hormones like cortisol.

6. The Alkaline Diet and Hormones:

- The alkaline diet emphasizes fruits, vegetables, nuts, and legumes, which are naturally alkalizing. This diet can help reduce inflammation and stress on the body, indirectly supporting hormonal health.

7. Individual Variations:

- Everyone's hormonal needs are different. Factors like age, gender, and health conditions affect how your diet impacts your hormones. Personalized nutrition is key.

Your diet is a powerful tool in maintaining hormonal balance. By choosing the right foods and understanding their impact, you can support your body's hormonal orchestra, leading to improved overall health and well-being.

Chapter 2

ALKALINE DIET
FUNDAMENTALS

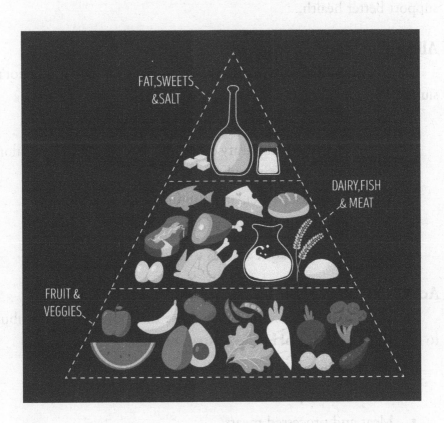

The alkaline diet, rooted in the idea that the foods we eat can affect the acidity or alkalinity of our bodies, isn't just a dietary choice—it's a lifestyle. The central premise is simple: by consuming more alkaline-forming foods and reducing acidic ones, we can improve our overall health. But what does this mean?

Understanding pH and Its Role

Our body's pH level, a scale measuring acidity and alkalinity, ranges from 0 (highly acidic) to 14 (highly alkaline), with 7 being neutral. Blood pH levels are tightly regulated by our bodies, typically staying around 7.4, slightly alkaline. The alkaline diet posits that by eating foods that promote a more alkaline environment in our bodies, we can support better health.

Alkaline Foods: What to Include

Alkaline-promoting foods are typically rich in minerals like potassium, calcium, and magnesium. These include:

- Fresh fruits like bananas, berries, and melons.
- Vegetables, especially leafy greens like spinach and kale, along with broccoli and cucumber.
- Nuts and seeds, particularly almonds and chia seeds.
- Whole grains, like quinoa and brown rice.
- Plant-based proteins, such as tofu and lentils.

Acidic Foods: What to Limit

On the flip side, acidic foods are those that potentially contribute to lowering the body's pH. These often include:

- Processed foods and sugars.
- Certain dairy products.
- Meat and processed meats.
- Caffeine and alcoholic beverages.

The Concept of Acid-Forming vs. Alkaline-Forming

It's crucial to distinguish between inherently acidic foods and those that have acid-forming effects on the body. For example, lemons are acidic but are considered alkaline-forming once metabolized.

Potential Health Benefits

Advocates of the alkaline diet claim numerous health benefits, such as:

- Improved bone health, as a less acidic environment, helps retain calcium.

- Enhanced kidney health, by reducing the strain on kidneys to maintain pH balance.

- Lowered risk for chronic diseases, based on the theory that an acidic environment promotes disease growth.

The Verdict: Balance is Key

While the idea of altering body pH through diet is debated, the alkaline diet's emphasis on whole foods and reduced processed food intake aligns with general healthy eating principles. The key takeaway? A balanced diet rich in fruits, vegetables, and whole grains, while limiting processed foods, supports overall health—whether you're strictly following the alkaline diet or just seeking a healthier lifestyle.

This overview of the alkaline diet fundamentals provides a clear understanding of its principles, food choices, and potential health benefits. The emphasis is on a balanced, healthful approach to eating, aligning with general nutritional guidelines.

THE PH SCALE AND OUR HEALTH

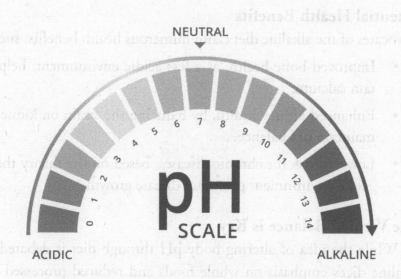

The pH scale, a concept often revisited in high school chemistry, is far more than just a scientific curiosity. It's a critical aspect of our health, profoundly impacting our body's functioning. This scale ranges from 0 to 14, with 7 being neutral. Numbers below 7 indicate acidity, while numbers above 7 denote alkalinity. Why does this matter for our health? Let's explore.

1. The Body's pH: A Delicate Balance

Our body works tirelessly to maintain a stable pH level, especially in the blood, where it hovers around a slightly alkaline level of 7.35 to 7.45. This balance is vital. Even minor deviations can disrupt bodily functions, affecting everything from digestion to immunity.

2. The Role of Diet

What we eat significantly influences our body's pH balance. Modern diets, heavy in processed foods, meat, and sugar, tend to be more acidic. This isn't ideal. Over time, an overly acidic diet can strain our body's regulatory systems. It's here the alkaline diet comes into play, emphasizing foods like fruits, vegetables, nuts, and legumes, known for their alkalizing effects.

3. Potential Health Benefits

Adopting an alkaline diet could bring several health benefits. Proponents suggest it can help maintain muscle mass, keep bones strong, and reduce the risk of chronic diseases. It's about creating an environment where the body thrives.

4. The Acid-Alkaline Myth

However, it's crucial to address a common misconception: the idea that you can drastically change your blood pH through diet. Our body regulates its pH so tightly that dietary changes won't cause significant shifts in blood pH. But, the diet's benefit lies in easing the body's regulatory burden and providing nutrient-rich foods.

5. A Holistic Approach

Focusing solely on pH can oversimplify health. It's not just about alkaline versus acidic foods. Balance is key. A healthy diet should include a variety of nutrients, regardless of their pH level.

6. Practical Application

How can we apply this knowledge? Start by incorporating more fruits and vegetables into your diet, reduce processed and high-sugar foods, and stay hydrated. It's about making conscious choices that support your body's natural balance.

In summary, while the pH scale is a fundamental concept, its role in diet and health is nuanced. An alkaline diet can contribute to overall well-being, but it should be part of a balanced, informed approach to health. Remember, no single food or diet is a magic bullet, but understanding and applying these principles can be a step toward better health.

Alkaline Foods

WHAT TO EAT FOR HORMONAL BALANCE

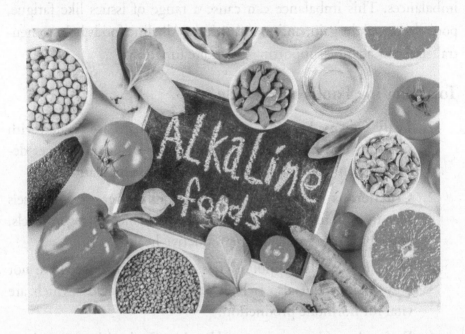

Alkaline foods play a crucial role in balancing hormones, which is essential for overall health and well-being, particularly for women. The concept is straightforward: certain foods can help maintain the body's optimal pH balance, leading to better hormonal health.

Understanding pH Balance

Firstly, let's delve into what pH balance means. The pH scale measures how acidic or alkaline something is, ranging from 0 to 14. A pH of 7 is neutral, below 7 is acidic, and above 7 is alkaline. The human body thrives when it maintains a slightly alkaline pH.

Why Alkaline Foods for Hormonal Balance?

Hormones, like insulin, cortisol, and estrogen, are sensitive to the body's pH level. When the body is too acidic, it can lead to hormonal imbalances. This imbalance can cause a range of issues like fatigue, poor sleep, weight gain, and mood swings. Alkaline foods help to neutralize excess acidity, supporting hormone function.

Top Alkaline Foods to Include

1. **Leafy Greens:** Spinach, kale, and Swiss chard are packed with nutrients and have high alkalinity. They are great for liver detoxification, which is essential for hormone regulation.

2. **Cruciferous Vegetables**: Broccoli, cauliflower, and Brussels sprouts contain compounds that help balance estrogen levels, crucial for menstrual and reproductive health.

3. **Nuts and Seeds:** Almonds, flaxseeds, and chia seeds are not only alkaline but also rich in omega-3 fatty acids, which are vital for hormone production.

4. **Fruits**: Avocado, coconut, and berries offer healthy fats and antioxidants while maintaining alkalinity. They also provide fiber, which aids digestion and hormone regulation.

5. **Root Vegetables:** Sweet potatoes, carrots, and beets are alkaline and provide complex carbohydrates and fiber, stabilizing blood sugar and insulin levels.

6. **Herbal Teas:** Herbal teas like ginger and peppermint are alkaline and can soothe the digestive system, further supporting hormonal balance.

Integrating Alkaline Foods into Your Diet

Incorporating these foods into your diet can be simple and delicious. Start by adding a serving of leafy greens to your meals, snack on nuts and seeds, and include a variety of colorful fruits and vegetables. Experiment with herbal teas to find flavors you enjoy.

Mindful Eating

It's not just about what you eat but also how you eat. Eating mindfully, chewing thoroughly, and not overeating can aid in digestion and absorption, which is beneficial for maintaining hormonal balance.

Balance is Key

Remember, balance is crucial. An overly alkaline diet isn't the goal. It's about creating a dietary balance that supports your body's natural pH level. Listen to your body and adjust as needed.

Alkaline foods offer a natural way to support hormonal health. By incorporating a variety of these foods into your diet, you can help maintain your body's pH balance, leading to improved hormonal function and overall health. Remember, every individual's body is different, so it's important to find the balance that works best for you.

Chapter 3

FOODS TO EMBRACE
AND AVOID

When it comes to managing hormonal health and adhering to an alkaline diet, the foods we eat play a pivotal role. Our diet can be our best ally in maintaining balance or our biggest challenge. This chapter offers an insightful guide into the world of foods, highlighting 50 items to embrace for their hormonal and alkaline benefits and 50 to avoid due to their adverse effects on hormonal balance and body pH levels.

Foods to Embrace

1. Spinach: Rich in magnesium, which aids in regulating cortisol levels.

2. Broccoli: Contains indole-3-carbinol, helping in estrogen balance.

3. Almonds: High in vitamin E, supporting hormonal health.

4. Avocados: Packed with healthy fats, promoting hormonal production.

5. Quinoa: A complete protein source, stabilizing blood sugar.

6. Sweet Potatoes: High in vitamin B6, crucial for progesterone balance.

7. Salmon: Rich in Omega-3s, reducing inflammation and supporting hormonal health.

8. Lemons: Alkaline-forming, helping to maintain the body's pH balance.

9. Turmeric: Contains curcumin, known for its anti-inflammatory properties.

10. Green Tea: Packed with antioxidants, promoting hormonal balance.

11. Kale: High in calcium, crucial for bone health during hormonal changes.

12. Chia Seeds: Rich in Omega-3 fatty acids, essential for hormonal health.

13. Flaxseeds: Contains lignans that help in balancing estrogen.

14. Walnuts: High in anti-inflammatory fats.

15. Coconut Oil: Provides healthy fats, aiding hormonal production.

16. Apple Cider Vinegar: Helps in maintaining alkaline pH levels.

17. Beets: Great for liver detoxification, which is essential for hormonal balance.

18. Garlic: Supports immune function and hormonal health.

19. Ginger: Anti-inflammatory and aids in digestion.

20. Pumpkin Seeds: Rich in zinc, important for hormone production.

21. Seaweed: High in iodine, crucial for thyroid health.

22. Asparagus: Great for liver detoxification and hormonal health.

23. Blueberries: Rich in antioxidants, supporting overall health.

24. Fermented Foods: Such as yogurt and kefir, for gut health.

25. Olive Oil: Healthy fat, important for hormone synthesis.

26. Pomegranate: Phytoestrogens can support hormonal balance.

27. Cinnamon: Helps regulate blood sugar levels.

28. Brussels Sprouts: Aid in detoxification and hormone regulation.

29. Sesame Seeds: High in calcium and phytoestrogens.

30. Eggs: Provide a complete protein source.

31. Lentils: High in fiber, supporting hormonal health.

32. Butternut Squash: High in vitamins and minerals.

33. Celery: Alkaline-forming and great for hydration.

34. Cucumbers: Help to maintain the body's alkaline pH.

35. Green Beans: Fiber-rich and supportive of hormonal health.

36. Tomatoes: Rich in lycopene, an antioxidant.

37. Mushrooms: Contain essential nutrients for hormonal health.

38. Carrots: High in fiber, supporting detoxification.

39. Red Bell Peppers: High in vitamin C, aiding adrenal health.

40. Zucchini: Good source of B vitamins.

41. Oats: Help stabilize blood sugar levels.

42. Bananas: High in potassium and B6, aiding hormonal balance.

43. Watercress: Alkaline-forming and nutrient-rich.

44. Parsley: Supports kidney health and hormonal balance.

45. Figs: Contain minerals that support hormonal health.

46. Kiwi: High in vitamins C and E.

47. Raspberries: Fiber-rich and support hormonal health.

48. Papaya: Enzymes in papaya aid in digestion.

49. Bok Choy: High in calcium, important for bone health.

50. Artichokes: Great for liver health and hormone balance.

Foods to Avoid

1. Sugar: This leads to hormonal imbalances and inflammation.
2. Refined Carbohydrates: Cause blood sugar spikes affecting hormones.
3. Caffeine: Can exacerbate hormonal imbalances.
4. Alcohol: Impacts liver function and hormonal balance.
5. Soy Products: High amounts can disrupt estrogen levels.
6. Processed Meats: Contain additives that can affect hormonal health.
7. High-Fructose Corn Syrup: Leads to insulin resistance.
8. Artificial Sweeteners: Can disrupt hormonal balance.
9. Trans Fats: Found in many processed foods, they disrupt hormone production.
10. Dairy Products: Can exacerbate hormonal imbalances in some women.
11. Gluten: For some, can cause inflammation affecting hormones.
12. Peanuts: May contain molds affecting hormonal health.
13. Conventional Meat: Hormones and antibiotics used can affect your hormonal balance.
14. Fried Foods: High in unhealthy fats, impacting hormonal health.
15. Canned Foods: Often contain BPA, which can act as an endocrine disruptor.

16. Energy Drinks: High caffeine and sugar content can disrupt hormones.

17. Non-Organic Fruits and Vegetables: Pesticides can affect hormonal balance.

18. Margarine: Often contains unhealthy trans fats.

19. Fast Food: High in unhealthy fats and chemicals.

20. White Bread: High glycemic index, affecting blood sugar levels.

21. Diet Sodas: Artificial sweeteners can disrupt hormonal balance.

22. Corn Oil: High in omega-6 fatty acids, can lead to inflammation.

23. Packaged Snacks: Often high in sugar and unhealthy fats.

24. Vegetable Shortening: High in trans fats.

25. Microwave Popcorn: Chemicals in the lining can disrupt hormones.

26. Conventional Dairy: Hormones and antibiotics can disrupt your own hormonal balance.

27. Farm-raised fish: Often contain pollutants and hormones.

28. Non-Organic Chicken: Hormones and antibiotics can affect hormonal health.

29. Agave Nectar: High in fructose, affecting insulin levels.

30. White Rice: High glycemic index, impacting blood sugar.

31. Table Salt: Processed and lacking minerals.

32. Soybean Oil: High in omega-6, can promote inflammation.

33. Instant Noodles: High in additives, low in nutrients.

34. Store-Bought Juices: High in sugar, low in fiber.

35. Pre-Packaged Meals: Often high in additives and preservatives.

36. Conventional Beef: Hormones and antibiotics can disrupt hormonal balance.

37. Flavored Yogurts: High in sugar, disrupting hormonal balance.

38. Artificial Flavors and Colors: Can be endocrine disruptors.

39. Canned Soup: High in sodium and often contains BPA.

40. Granola Bars: Often high in sugar and unhealthy fats.

41. Bottled Salad Dressings: High in unhealthy fats and sugars.

42. Conventional Apples: Pesticides can affect hormonal health.

43. Potato Chips: High in unhealthy fats and salts.

44. Non-Organic Potatoes: High pesticide residue.

45. Ice Cream: High in sugar and often contains additives.

46. Non-Organic Strawberries: High pesticide residue.

47. Pre-Packaged Baked Goods: High in trans fats and sugars.

48. Non-Organic Grapes: Pesticides can disrupt hormonal balance.

49. Instant Coffee: Often contains added chemicals.

50. Artificial Creamers: High in unhealthy fats and chemicals.

By understanding the foods that support hormonal balance and those that hinder it, women can make empowered choices to nurture their bodies and maintain their well-being.

SUPERFOODS FOR HORMONAL HEALTH

Hormonal balance is like a symphony in our bodies—each hormone must play its part perfectly for overall harmony. And, just like a symphony needs the right instruments, our hormones need the right nutrients to perform optimally. This is where superfoods come in, offering a powerhouse of essential nutrients that are particularly beneficial for women's hormonal health.

1. Cruciferous Vegetables: Broccoli, Cauliflower, and Brussels Sprouts

These aren't just your ordinary greens. Cruciferous vegetables are champions in balancing estrogen levels. They contain a compound called indole-3-carbinol which, when digested, forms diindolylmethane (DIM). DIM plays a crucial role in metabolizing estrogen, ensuring it's broken down into beneficial rather than harmful forms. This can be particularly beneficial in reducing the risk of estrogen-related conditions like breast cancer.

2. Fatty Fish: Salmon, Mackerel, and Sardines

Rich in Omega-3 fatty acids, fatty fish are a boon for hormonal health. Omega-3s help reduce inflammation, which is crucial since chronic inflammation can disrupt hormonal signaling. Additionally, these fats are essential for the production of hormones and can aid in balancing mood-related hormones, reducing the symptoms of PMS and menopause.

3. Seeds: Flaxseeds and Chia Seeds

Seeds might be small, but their impact on hormonal health is significant. Flaxseeds are particularly noteworthy for their phytoestrogens, which mimic estrogen in the body and can help balance hormone levels. They are also high in fiber, which aids in hormone excretion. Chia seeds, on the other hand, are packed with Omega-3s and fiber, supporting overall hormonal health.

4. Nuts: Almonds and Walnuts

Nuts, especially almonds and walnuts, are great for hormonal health. They're packed with magnesium, a mineral that plays a critical role in hormone production. Magnesium can help regulate cortisol (the stress hormone), thus aiding in stress management. Moreover, almonds contain vitamin E, which can alleviate PMS symptoms.

5. Avocado

Avocado is more than a trendy brunch staple. It's a hormonal health superstar. Rich in healthy fats, avocados support overall endocrine function. They also contain beta-sitosterol, which can have a balancing effect on cortisol levels, helping to reduce stress.

6. Leafy Greens: Spinach and Kale

Leafy greens like spinach and kale are high in magnesium and iron, two minerals essential for healthy hormone function. Iron is particularly important for women who experience heavy menstrual cycles, as it helps prevent anemia, a condition that can exacerbate hormonal imbalance.

7. Berries: Blueberries and Strawberries

Berries are not only delicious but also packed with antioxidants. These compounds help protect cells from damage and reduce inflammation, which is crucial for maintaining hormonal balance. The natural sweetness of berries can also help curb sugar cravings, which is beneficial for maintaining a steady blood sugar level.

8. Quinoa

This gluten-free grain is a complete protein, containing all nine essential amino acids. Proteins are the building blocks for hormones, making quinoa an excellent food for hormonal health. It also has a high magnesium content, further supporting hormonal balance.

9. Fermented Foods: Yogurt, Kefir, and Sauerkraut

Fermented foods are rich in probiotics, beneficial bacteria that play a crucial role in gut health. A healthy gut is essential for hormone balance, as it aids in the elimination of excess hormones and the absorption of nutrients needed for hormone production.

10. Dark Chocolate

Yes, even chocolate can be a superfood when it comes to hormones! Dark chocolate (at least 70% cocoa) is rich in magnesium and flavonoids. It can help boost mood and alleviate stress, making it a delightful addition to a hormonal health diet.

TOP FOODS THAT DISRUPT
HORMONAL BALANCE

When it comes to maintaining a healthy hormonal balance, what we eat plays a pivotal role. While some foods can support and enhance hormonal function, others can disrupt it. Understanding these disruptors is crucial, especially for women, as hormonal imbalances can lead to a range of health issues, from menstrual irregularities to mood swings, weight gain, and more.

1. Processed and Sugary Foods

- The Sugar Trap: Consuming high amounts of sugar and processed foods can lead to insulin resistance. Insulin is a hormone that regulates blood sugar levels. When your body starts resisting insulin's effects, it can lead to conditions like type 2 diabetes and polycystic ovary syndrome (PCOS).

- The Blood Sugar Rollercoaster: These foods cause rapid spikes and drops in blood sugar levels, which can disrupt the balance of other hormones like cortisol (the stress hormone) and estrogen.

2. High-Caffeine Beverages

- The Caffeine Effect: While a small amount of caffeine can be energizing, excessive consumption, especially in the form of coffee and energy drinks, can overstimulate the adrenal glands. This overstimulation can lead to an imbalance in cortisol production, impacting stress levels, sleep quality, and overall hormonal health.

3. Dairy Products

- Hormones in Dairy: Many dairy products contain hormones that are naturally present in the animals. These external hormones can mimic our own hormones, potentially leading to imbalances.

- Dairy Sensitivity: Some women may also have a sensitivity to dairy, which can trigger inflammatory responses, further exacerbating hormonal imbalances.

4. Soy Products

- Phytoestrogens: Soy contains phytoestrogens, compounds that can mimic the hormone estrogen in the body. While moderate consumption may be beneficial for some, excessive intake can disrupt the delicate balance of estrogen and progesterone, especially in women with estrogen-dominance conditions.

5. Alcohol

- Impact on Liver Function: Regular consumption of alcohol can impact liver function. The liver plays a key role in hormone regulation by metabolizing hormones. An overworked liver can lead to an accumulation of hormones, particularly estrogen, leading to imbalances.

- Interference with Sleep and Stress: Alcohol can also interfere with sleep quality and increase stress levels, both of which are vital for maintaining hormonal balance.

6. Refined Carbohydrates

- Insulin Spikes: Foods like white bread, pastries, and other refined carbs can cause sudden spikes in insulin levels, similar to sugary foods. Over time, this can lead to insulin resistance and hormonal imbalances.

7. Trans Fats and Hydrogenated Oils

- Inflammatory Response: These unhealthy fats, often found in fried and processed foods, can trigger an inflammatory response in the body. Inflammation is a known disruptor of hormonal balance and can exacerbate conditions like endometriosis and menstrual pain.

Avoiding these foods is not about strict prohibitions but rather about creating a balanced diet that supports your hormonal health. It's about making informed choices. Maybe it's choosing a piece of fruit over a candy bar, or water over a sugary drink. These small decisions can add up to a significant impact on your overall hormonal health.

Remember, every woman's body is unique. What disrupts hormonal balance in one person may not have the same effect in another. Listening to your body is key. If you suspect certain foods are affecting your hormonal balance, consider talking to a nutritionist or healthcare provider. They can provide personalized advice based on your individual health needs.

Chapter 4

PLANNING YOUR HORMONAL HEALTH DIET

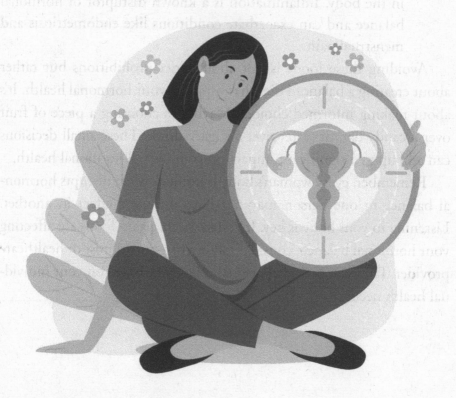

Understanding Your Body's Needs

Every woman's body is unique, and so are her dietary needs. It's not just about eating healthy; it's about understanding what your body specifically requires to maintain hormonal balance. Start with a health check-up. Knowing your baseline hormone levels, blood sugar, and nutrient deficiencies is crucial.

Key Nutrients for Hormonal Health

1. Healthy Fats: These are vital for hormone production. Avocados, nuts, and seeds are great sources.

2. Fiber: It helps in digestion and regulating blood sugar levels. Think whole grains, legumes, and vegetables.

3. Protein: Essential for muscle repair and hormone synthesis. Lean meats, fish, and plant-based proteins like quinoa and lentils are excellent choices.

4. Cruciferous Vegetables: Broccoli, cauliflower, and Brussels sprouts support liver function and hormonal detoxification.

The Alkaline Touch

An alkaline diet emphasizes foods that help maintain a healthy pH level in the body. It's not about completely avoiding acidic foods but finding the right balance. Alkaline foods include most fruits and vegetables, nuts, and seeds. A simple tip is to fill half your plate with vegetables at each meal.

Meal Planning

Plan your meals. This doesn't mean you need a rigid menu but having a general idea helps in maintaining a balanced diet. For instance, plan to have fish twice a week, a vegetarian meal on Wednesdays, and so on.

Listening to Your Body

Pay attention to how different foods make you feel. Does dairy make you feel bloated? Do you feel energetic after eating a high-protein meal? Adjust your diet accordingly. Remember, this is a journey to understand and cater to your body's unique needs.

Sample Meal Ideas

1. Breakfast: A smoothie with spinach, a banana, almond milk, and a scoop of protein powder.

2. Lunch: Quinoa salad with chickpeas, cucumber, tomatoes, and a lemon-olive oil dressing.

3. Dinner: Grilled salmon with steamed broccoli and a side of sweet potato.

Snacking Smartly

Choose snacks that support your hormonal health. Greek yogurt, a handful of almonds, or carrot sticks with hummus are great choices. Avoid processed foods as much as possible.

Hydration

Don't forget about water! Staying hydrated is essential for overall health and helps in detoxification.

Supplements

While getting nutrients from food is ideal, sometimes supplements are necessary, especially if you have specific deficiencies. Consult with a healthcare provider before starting any supplement.

Conclusion

Embarking on a hormonal health diet isn't about drastic changes overnight. It's about making mindful choices, understanding your body, and gradually adopting a lifestyle that supports your hormonal health. Remember, the goal is balance, not perfection.

MEAL PLANNING AND PREPARATION

Understanding the Basics

Meal planning and preparation are cornerstones of maintaining a balanced hormonal and alkaline diet. It's not just about choosing the right foods; it's about creating a sustainable routine that supports your hormonal health.

The Importance of Planning

1. **Efficiency and Time Management:** Planning your meals for the week can save you time and reduce stress. No more last-minute scrambles or unhealthy choices due to lack of preparation.
2. **Balanced Nutrient Intake:** By planning, you ensure that each meal is balanced and contributes to your overall nutritional needs, crucial for hormonal balance.
3. **Budget-Friendly:** Planned meals reduce impulsive purchases and food waste, helping you manage your grocery budget more effectively.

Key Considerations in Meal Planning

1. **Hormonal Needs:** Women's bodies require different nutrients at various stages of their menstrual cycle. For instance, magnesium and B vitamins might be more beneficial during the premenstrual phase.
2. **Alkalinity:** Focus on including alkaline foods like fruits, vegetables, nuts, and seeds. These help maintain a healthy pH balance in the body, which is vital for hormonal equilibrium.

3. **Diversity in Diet:** Ensure your meal plan includes a variety of foods. This not only keeps meals interesting but also ensures a wide range of nutrients.

Meal Preparation Tips

1. **Batch Cooking:** Cook in large quantities and store in portions. This strategy works well for grains, proteins, and vegetables.
2. **Smart Snacking:** Prepare healthy snacks in advance. Think cut veggies, fruit slices, or a handful of almonds. These are great for keeping hunger at bay and maintaining stable blood sugar levels.
3. **Simplifying Recipes:** Choose recipes that are easy to make and don't require rare ingredients. The simpler it is, the more likely you'll stick to it.

Incorporating Superfoods

1. **Leafy Greens:** Spinach, kale, and Swiss chard are excellent for an alkaline diet.
2. **Seeds and Nuts:** Chia seeds, flaxseeds, and almonds are not only alkaline but also rich in essential fatty acids which are great for hormonal health.
3. **Berries and Citrus Fruits:** These are high in antioxidants and vitamins, supporting overall health and providing necessary dietary fiber.

Examples of Hormonal and Alkaline Diet Meals

1. **Breakfast:** A smoothie with spinach, banana, almond milk, and a scoop of protein powder.
2. **Lunch:** Quinoa salad with mixed greens, cherry tomatoes,

cucumber, and a lemon-olive oil dressing.

3. **Dinner:** Grilled salmon with steamed broccoli and sweet potato.

Listening to Your Body

Always pay attention to how your body reacts to certain foods. Personalization is key in a hormonal and alkaline diet. What works for one may not work for another.

Remember, the goal of meal planning in a hormonal and alkaline diet is not just about strict dietary restrictions. It's about creating a harmonious relationship with food that supports your hormonal health, keeps your body in balance, and fits into your lifestyle seamlessly. With thoughtful planning and preparation, you can make this diet a sustainable and enjoyable part of your life.

30-DAY HORMONAL AND ALKALINE DIET MEAL PLAN

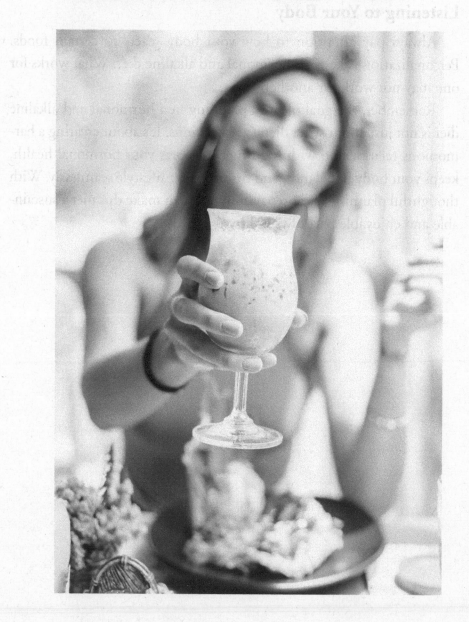

Day 1

- **Breakfast**: Spinach and feta omelet with whole-grain toast
- **Lunch**: Quinoa and chickpea salad with cucumber, tomatoes, and lemon vinaigrette
- **Dinner**: Grilled chicken breast with steamed asparagus and wild rice

Day 2

- **Breakfast**: Greek yogurt with mixed berries and a sprinkle of chia seeds
- **Lunch**: Turkey and avocado wrap with whole-grain tortilla, lettuce, and tomato
- Dinner: Baked salmon with a side of roasted Brussels sprouts and sweet potato

Day 3

- **Breakfast**: Smoothie with almond milk, banana, spinach, and protein powder
- **Lunch**: Lentil soup with a side of mixed greens salad
- **Dinner**: Stir-fried tofu with broccoli, bell peppers, and brown rice

Day 4

- **Breakfast**: Scrambled eggs with kale and mushrooms
- **Lunch**: Tuna salad with mixed greens, avocado, and olive oil dressing
- **Dinner**: Beef stir-fry with quinoa and a variety of vegetables

Day 5

- **Breakfast**: Oatmeal with sliced almonds and blueberries
- **Lunch**: Grilled chicken Caesar salad with romaine lettuce and a yogurt-based dressing
- **Dinner**: Baked cod with a side of quinoa and steamed green beans

Day 6

- **Breakfast**: Protein pancakes topped with fresh strawberries
- **Lunch**: Chickpea and vegetable curry with brown rice
- **Dinner**: Grilled shrimp with a mixed vegetable medley and couscous

Day 7

- **Breakfast**: Avocado toast on whole-grain bread with poached eggs
- **Lunch**: Roasted vegetable and feta cheese salad
- **Dinner**: Lemon garlic baked chicken with a side of roasted root vegetables

Day 8

- **Breakfast**: Chia seed pudding made with almond milk, topped with sliced banana, and a sprinkle of cinnamon.
- **Lunch**: Grilled vegetable and quinoa salad with a lemon-tahini dressing.
- **Dinner**: Lemon-herb roasted chicken with a side of steamed broccoli and carrots.

Day 9

- **Breakfast**: Whole-grain toast with almond butter and sliced apple.
- **Lunch**: Lentil and vegetable stew with a side of mixed green salad.
- **Dinner**: Baked trout with a side of sautéed spinach and roasted butternut squash.

Day 10

- **Breakfast**: Green smoothie with kale, pineapple, avocado, and ginger.
- **Lunch**: Turkey and cranberry salad with mixed greens and balsamic vinaigrette.
- **Dinner**: Stir-fried beef with bell peppers, broccoli, and brown rice.

Day 11

- **Breakfast**: Cottage cheese with fresh peaches and a sprinkle of flax seeds.
- **Lunch**: Grilled chicken and avocado wrap with a whole-grain tortilla.
- **Dinner**: Vegetarian chili with kidney beans, tomatoes, and a variety of vegetables, served with brown rice.

Day 12

- **Breakfast**: Omelet with spinach, tomatoes, and mushrooms.
- **Lunch**: Baked falafel with a quinoa tabbouleh salad.

- **Dinner**: Grilled salmon with a side of asparagus and a quinoa pilaf.

Day 13

- **Breakfast**: Berry and yogurt parfait with a layer of granola.
- **Lunch**: Roasted beet and goat cheese salad with walnuts.
- **Dinner**: Chicken curry with mixed vegetables and basmati rice.

Day 14

- **Breakfast**: Overnight oats with almond milk, chia seeds, and mixed berries.
- **Lunch**: Tuna and white bean salad with a light lemon dressing.
- **Dinner**: Shrimp stir-fry with snap peas, bell peppers, and brown rice noodles.

Day 15

- **Breakfast**: Banana and walnut muffins made with almond flour.
- **Lunch**: Avocado and black bean salad with corn, tomatoes, and cilantro.
- **Dinner**: Baked cod with a Mediterranean tomato and olive topping, served with steamed green beans.

Day 16

- **Breakfast**: Greek yogurt with granola and a drizzle of honey.
- **Lunch**: Quinoa stuffed bell peppers with a side of mixed greens.
- **Dinner**: Garlic and herb grilled chicken with a side of roasted Brussels sprouts and a sweet potato.

Day 17

- **Breakfast**: Smoothie bowl with spinach, banana, mixed berries, and a sprinkle of hemp seeds.
- **Lunch**: Lentil salad with cucumbers, tomatoes, feta, and a lemon-olive oil dressing.
- **Dinner**: Baked tilapia with a side of steamed vegetables and wild rice.

Day 18

- **Breakfast**: Whole grain toast with avocado and poached eggs.
- **Lunch**: Chicken and vegetable soup with a side of whole-grain bread.
- **Dinner**: Veggie stir-fry with tofu, broccoli, carrots, and brown rice.

Day 19

- **Breakfast**: Berry and spinach smoothie with almond milk and a scoop of protein powder.
- **Lunch**: Turkey, avocado, and spinach wrapped in a whole-grain tortilla.
- **Dinner**: Grilled shrimp skewers with a quinoa and vegetable salad.

Day 20

- **Breakfast**: Oatmeal with sliced banana, walnuts, and a dash of cinnamon.
- **Lunch**: Mediterranean chickpea salad with olives, cucumber,

and feta.

- **Dinner**: Lemon pepper baked salmon with asparagus and a side of quinoa.

Day 21

- **Breakfast**: Scrambled eggs with sautéed mushrooms, spinach, and tomatoes.
- **Lunch**: Caprese salad with fresh mozzarella, tomatoes, basil, and a balsamic glaze.
- **Dinner**: Beef and vegetable kebabs with a side of couscous.

Day 22

- **Breakfast**: Protein pancakes topped with fresh berries and a dollop of Greek yogurt.
- **Lunch**: Tuna salad served over a bed of mixed greens.
- **Dinner**: Vegetarian curry with chickpeas, spinach, and sweet potatoes, served with brown rice.

Day 23

- **Breakfast**: Chia pudding made with coconut milk, topped with mango and coconut flakes.
- **Lunch**: Roasted chicken salad with mixed greens, avocado, and cherry tomatoes.
- **Dinner**: Baked haddock with a side of roasted cauliflower and a mixed bean salad.

Day 24

- **Breakfast**: Almond butter and banana smoothie with a scoop of protein powder.

- **Lunch**: Quinoa bowl with black beans, corn, bell peppers, and a lime cilantro dressing.

- **Dinner**: Lemon and herb roasted turkey breast with steamed green beans and a side of wild rice.

Day 25

- **Breakfast**: Whole-grain toast with smoked salmon, cream cheese, and cucumber.

- **Lunch**: Beetroot and goat cheese salad with walnuts and a side of sourdough bread.

- **Dinner**: Grilled lamb chops with a mint yogurt sauce, served with a side of roasted Mediterranean vegetables.

Day 26

- **Breakfast**: Greek yogurt with granola and mixed berries.

- **Lunch**: Turkey and cranberry sandwich on whole-grain bread with a side of carrot sticks.

- **Dinner**: Stir-fried shrimp with broccoli, carrots, and snow peas, served over brown rice.

Day 27

- **Breakfast**: Oatmeal with almond milk, topped with sliced peaches and a drizzle of honey.

- **Lunch**: Spinach and feta stuffed chicken breast with a side of quinoa tabbouleh.

- **Dinner**: Baked cod with a lemon butter sauce, served with steamed asparagus and a sweet potato mash.

Day 28

- **Breakfast**: Scrambled tofu with spinach, bell peppers, and onions.

- **Lunch**: Avocado and chicken Caesar salad with a   yogurt-based dressing.

- **Dinner**: Beef stir-fry with mixed vegetables and a side of quinoa.

Day 29

- **Breakfast**: Protein shake with spinach, blueberries, and almond milk.

- **Lunch**: Mediterranean chickpea and vegetable wrap in a whole-grain tortilla.

- **Dinner**: Grilled pork chops with a side of apple slaw and roasted Brussels sprouts.

Day 30

- **Breakfast**: Cottage cheese with pineapple chunks and a sprinkle of sunflower seeds.

- **Lunch**: Rainbow vegetable noodle salad with a ginger sesame dressing.

- **Dinner**: Roasted duck breast with a balsamic glaze, served with a side of wild rice pilaf and steamed green beans.

NOTE:

Snacks (Choose 2 Daily):

- A handful of nuts (almonds, walnuts)
- Fresh fruit (apples, oranges, berries)
- Vegetable sticks with hummus
- Greek yogurt with a drizzle of honey
- A small portion of dark chocolate

ADDITIONAL TIPS:

- Adaptability: The meal plan is a guideline and can be adjusted to suit individual tastes, dietary needs, and nutritional goals.

- Portion Size: Be mindful of portions to maintain a balanced diet.

- Seasonal and Fresh: Where possible, use seasonal and fresh ingredients for maximum nutritional benefits.

- Stay Hydrated: Alongside meals, ensure adequate water intake.

- Mindful Eating: Pay attention to your body's hunger and fullness cues. Eating mindfully helps in better digestion and hormonal balance.

RECIPE SAMPLES FOR HORMONAL BALANCE AND ALKALINITY

Breakfast

AVOCADO AND SPINACH SMOOTHIE

- Prep Time: 5 minutes
- Serves: 1
- Nutrition Per Serving: Calories: 220, Protein: 4g, Carbohydrates: 18g, Fat: 15g, Fiber: 7g

Ingredients:

- 1 ripe avocado
- 1 cup fresh spinach
- 1 banana
- 1/2 cup almond milk (unsweetened)
- 1 tbsp chia seeds
- 1 tsp honey (optional)
- Ice cubes (optional)

Directions:

1. Cut the avocado in half, remove the pit, and scoop out the flesh.
2. In a blender, combine the avocado, spinach, banana, almond milk, chia seeds, and honey if using. Add ice cubes for a colder smoothie.
3. Blend until smooth and creamy.
4. Pour into a glass and enjoy immediately.

Lunch

QUINOA AND ROASTED VEGETABLE SALAD

- Prep Time: 30 minutes
- Serves: 2
- Nutrition Per Serving: Calories: 310, Protein: 9g, Carbohydrates: 45g, Fat: 12g, Fiber: 8g

Ingredients:

- 1 cup quinoa
- 2 cups water
- 1 red bell pepper, chopped
- 1 zucchini, sliced
- 1 small red onion, chopped
- 2 tbsp olive oil
- Salt and pepper, to taste
- 2 tbsp lemon juice
- 1/4 cup chopped fresh parsley

Directions:

1. Preheat the oven to 400°F (200°C).
2. In a pot, bring the quinoa and water to a boil, then simmer for 15-20 minutes until the quinoa is cooked.
3. Toss the bell pepper, zucchini, and red onion with olive oil, salt, and pepper. Spread on a baking sheet.

Dinner

GRILLED SALMON WITH
STEAMED ASPARAGUS

- Prep Time: 20 minutes
- Serves: 2
- Nutrition Per Serving: Calories: 345, Protein: 35g, Carbohydrates: 5g, Fat: 20g, Fiber: 2g

Ingredients:

- 2 salmon fillets (about 6 oz each)
- 1 tbsp olive oil
- Salt and pepper, to taste
- 1 bunch asparagus, ends trimmed
- Lemon wedges, for serving

Directions:

1. Preheat the grill to medium-high heat.
2. Brush the salmon with olive oil and season with salt and pepper.
3. Grill the salmon for 5-6 minutes on each side, or until cooked through.
4. Meanwhile, steam the asparagus for 3-4 minutes until tender but still crisp.
5. Serve the salmon and asparagus with lemon wedges.

4. Roast the vegetables for 20 minutes, stirring halfway.

5. Mix the cooked quinoa with roasted vegetables, lemon juice, and parsley.

6. Serve warm or at room temperature.

Dessert

BAKED APPLE WITH CINNAMON AND NUTS

- Prep Time: 40 minutes
- Serves: 2
- Nutrition Per Serving: Calories: 190, Protein: 2g, Carbohydrates: 35g, Fat: 6g, Fiber: 5g

Ingredients:
- 2 large apples
- 1/4 cup chopped walnuts
- 2 tsp cinnamon
- 1 tbsp honey
- 1/4 cup water

Directions:
1. Preheat the oven to 350°F (175°C).
2. Core the apples and place them in a baking dish.
3. Mix the walnuts, cinnamon, and honey. Stuff this mixture into the apples.
4. Pour water into the bottom of the dish.
5. Bake for 30 minutes, or until the apples are tender.

Snack

HUMMUS AND VEGGIE STICKS

- Prep Time: 10 minutes
- Serves: 2
- Nutrition Per Serving: Calories: 150, Protein: 6g, Carbohydrates: 20g, Fat: 6g, Fiber: 5g

Ingredients:

- 1 cup homemade or store-bought hummus
- 1 carrot, cut into sticks
- 1 cucumber, cut into sticks
- 1 bell pepper, cut into sticks

Directions:

1. Arrange the hummus in a small bowl.
2. Serve with carrot, cucumber, and bell pepper sticks for dipping.

These recipes are designed to balance hormones and maintain an alkaline diet, using fresh, wholesome ingredients. Each recipe provides a good mix of nutrients while being simple and enjoyable to prepare and eat.

Chapter 5

UNDERSTANDING YOUR
BODY'S SIGNALS

Our bodies are constantly communicating with us, often through subtle signs and signals. When it comes to hormonal health, these signals can be particularly telling. They might manifest as mood swings, unexplained weight gain or loss, fatigue, or even changes in skin condition. It's essential to become attuned to these messages. For example, persistent fatigue might be more than just a lack of sleep; it could be a sign of hormonal imbalance.

The Role of Diet in Hormonal Signals

What we eat has a profound impact on our hormonal health. Foods high in sugar and processed ingredients can cause spikes in insulin and stress hormones, leading to a host of issues like inflammation and hormonal imbalances. On the flip side, a diet rich in whole, alkaline foods can support hormonal balance. Alkaline diets, which emphasize fruits, vegetables, nuts, and seeds, help maintain the body's ideal pH level, fostering an environment where hormones can function optimally.

Listening to Hunger and Fullness Cues

Understanding hunger and fullness cues is crucial. Sometimes, what we perceive as hunger can be a signal of dehydration or nutritional deficiency. Learning to differentiate these cues can guide us toward healthier eating habits. Similarly, overeating or emotional eating can be a response to hormonal imbalances. A diet that balances hormones will often lead to more natural hunger cues.

The Impact of Stress and Sleep

Stress and sleep are closely linked to hormonal health. Chronic stress can lead to elevated cortisol levels, disrupting sleep and other hormonal functions. Conversely, inadequate sleep can lead to imbalances in hormones like leptin and ghrelin, which regulate appetite. Recognizing these patterns can help in adopting strategies, such as mindfulness and adequate sleep hygiene, to maintain hormonal balance.

Physical Symptoms to Watch For

Physical symptoms like irregular menstrual cycles, digestive issues, and changes in hair and skin can be key indicators of hormonal imbalances. Keeping a symptom diary can be a helpful way to track these changes and discuss them with a healthcare provider.

Emotional and Cognitive Signals

Emotional and cognitive changes are also critical to note. Hormonal imbalances can manifest as anxiety, depression, or brain fog. Understanding the link between diet, hormone levels, and mental health is essential. Nutrients from an alkaline diet can support brain health and mood regulation.

Intuitive Eating and Mindful Nutrition

Intuitive eating is about listening to your body's natural hunger and fullness signals. It's a practice that aligns well with maintaining hormonal balance. Mindful nutrition involves being aware of how foods affect your mood and energy levels and making dietary choices that support your overall well-being.

In conclusion, understanding our body's signals is a journey of tuning in to its unique needs and responses. By paying attention to these cues, particularly in the context of a hormonal and alkaline diet, women can embark on a path toward improved health and wellness. This chapter aims to empower readers with the knowledge to interpret these signals and make informed decisions about their health.

RECOGNIZING HORMONAL IMBALANCES

In our journey to understand the delicate balance of the human body, especially for women, recognizing hormonal imbalances is a critical step. Hormones are like your body's internal messengers; they travel in your bloodstream to tissues and organs, delivering messages that control many of your body's major processes. When these hormonal levels are out of balance, it's like having a miscommunication in your body's messaging system. This can lead to a range of symptoms, some subtle and others more pronounced.

Common Signs of Hormonal Imbalance

1. Irregular Menstrual Cycles: One of the most straightforward indicators of hormonal issues is the menstrual cycle. If your cycles are irregular, too long, too short, or absent, it might be a sign of hormonal imbalance.

2. Unexplained Weight Changes: A sudden weight change, especially without a change in diet or exercise habits, can be a sign of hormonal issues. Both weight gain and loss can be relevant.

3. Mood Swings and Mental Health Fluctuations: Hormones significantly influence mental health. Feelings of anxiety, depression, or irritability that seem to come out of nowhere might be linked to hormonal shifts.

4. Fatigue: Constantly feeling tired, regardless of how much you sleep, can also indicate an imbalance, particularly involving thyroid hormones.

5. Sleep Problems: Difficulty falling asleep or staying asleep can be linked to hormonal imbalances, especially those involving

progesterone and estrogen.

6. Skin and Hair Changes: Acne, dry skin, or hair loss can also be a symptom of hormonal changes.

Understanding the Causes

While it's normal for hormone levels to fluctuate over a woman's life, certain conditions and lifestyle factors can exacerbate these imbalances:

- Stress: Chronic stress can wreak havoc on your hormones, particularly cortisol and adrenaline.

- Poor Diet and Nutrition: A diet lacking in essential nutrients can affect hormonal function. This is where an alkaline diet, rich in whole, unprocessed foods, can play a significant role.

- Lack of Exercise: Regular physical activity helps to regulate hormones.

- Environmental Factors: Exposure to certain chemicals and pollutants can disrupt hormonal balance.

The Role of Diet in Balancing Hormones

An alkaline diet, which emphasizes fresh fruits, vegetables, nuts, and seeds, can be instrumental in restoring hormonal balance. These foods are not only nutrient-rich but also help maintain a healthy pH level in the body, which is essential for optimal hormonal function. For instance, leafy greens are rich in magnesium, a mineral that plays a crucial role in the production of hormones.

When to Seek Professional Help

It's important to listen to your body. If you suspect a hormonal imbalance, it's advisable to consult with a healthcare professional. They can conduct appropriate tests to confirm hormonal imbalances and guide you on the right course of treatment, which may include dietary changes, lifestyle modifications, or medical interventions.

In summary, recognizing the signs of hormonal imbalances is the first step toward taking control of your health. By understanding these symptoms and their causes, and considering the role of a balanced diet, like the alkaline diet, women can take proactive steps towards maintaining their hormonal health. Remember, every woman's body is unique, and what works for one may not work for another. Therefore, it's crucial to approach hormonal health as a personalized journey.

THE ROLE OF DIET IN MANAGING SYMPTOMS

Understanding the Connection

The foods we eat can have a profound impact on our hormonal balance, which in turn affects our overall health and well-being. Hormones, like insulin, estrogen, and cortisol, are chemical messengers that play a crucial role in regulating bodily functions. When these are out of balance, it can lead to a variety of symptoms, such as fatigue, weight gain, mood swings, and even more serious health conditions.

Hormonal Imbalance and Diet

A diet high in processed foods, sugar, and unhealthy fats can contribute to hormonal imbalance. These foods can cause spikes in insulin levels, increase inflammation, and disrupt your gut health, which is crucial for hormone regulation. On the other hand, a balanced diet rich in whole foods can help maintain hormonal equilibrium.

Alkaline Diet: A Key Player

The alkaline diet focuses on foods that help maintain the body's ideal pH level. This diet emphasizes fruits, vegetables, nuts, and seeds, all of which are not only alkaline-forming but also rich in nutrients that support hormonal health. For example, leafy greens are high in magnesium, a mineral that plays a critical role in the production of hormone-regulating enzymes.

Specific Foods for Symptom Management

- For Estrogen Balance: Include foods like flaxseeds, which contain phytoestrogens that can help balance estrogen levels.

- To Support Thyroid Function: Foods rich in iodine, like seaweed, are vital as the thyroid uses iodine to make hormones.

- For Adrenal Health: Foods high in vitamin C and B vitamins, such as citrus fruits and whole grains, can support adrenal glands that produce stress hormones.

Inflammation and Hormones

Inflammation is a key factor in hormonal imbalance. An alkaline diet, rich in anti-inflammatory foods like omega-3 fatty acids found in fish and chia seeds, can help reduce inflammation and thereby support hormonal health.

Gut Health and Hormones

A healthy gut is essential for hormone balance. Probiotic-rich foods like yogurt and fermented vegetables can improve gut health, aiding in hormone regulation and symptom management.

Lifestyle Integration

Diet alone isn't a silver bullet. It works best when combined with a healthy lifestyle that includes regular exercise, stress management, and adequate sleep. All these factors work synergistically to manage symptoms and promote hormonal balance.

In summary, your diet plays a pivotal role in managing symptoms related to hormonal imbalances. By focusing on an alkaline diet and incorporating specific foods that support hormone health, you can significantly improve your symptoms and overall well-being. Remember, it's not about a quick fix, but rather a sustainable lifestyle change that supports your body's natural balance.

Chapter 6

LIFESTYLE AND BEYOND DIET

Exercise and Hormonal Health

Starting with exercise, it's not just about losing weight or building strength; it's deeply intertwined with your hormonal health. Regular physical activity can significantly impact your hormones, from reducing insulin resistance to boosting mood-enhancing endorphins. For instance, aerobic exercises, like brisk walking or cycling, can help increase insulin sensitivity, which is vital for hormonal balance. Resistance training, on the other hand, can enhance muscle strength and metabolism. But here's the key – it's not about intense workouts every day. Consistency and moderation are your best friends. Overdoing it can stress your body and throw your hormones off balance.

Stress Management

Now, let's talk about stress. It's like that uninvited guest at a party who just won't leave. Chronic stress can wreak havoc on your hormonal balance, leading to issues like adrenal fatigue, where your cortisol levels are all over the place. How do you combat this? Through techniques like mindfulness, meditation, and deep breathing exercises. These practices don't just sound calming; they have a profound physiological impact, helping to lower cortisol levels and improve your overall hormonal health.

The Importance of Sleep

Moving on to sleep – it's not just a luxury; it's a necessity. Lack of sleep can mess with your hormones, especially cortisol and insulin. Aim for 7-8 hours of quality sleep per night. Establish a regular sleep schedule, create a bedtime routine, and make your bedroom a sanctuary for rest. Remember, good sleep hygiene can be a game-changer for hormonal balance.

Environmental Factors

Don't forget the environment around you. Daily exposure to toxins, whether it's from plastic containers, non-stick cookware, or even your shampoo, can introduce hormone disruptors into your body. Start by making small changes like switching to glass containers or choosing paraben-free personal care products. Every little bit helps in reducing your exposure to these endocrine disruptors.

Social Connections and Mental Health

Lastly, your social life and mental health are pivotal. Strong social connections can boost your emotional well-being and, in turn, positively influence your hormones. Engage in activities that bring joy and connect you with others. And if you're feeling overwhelmed, never hesitate to seek support from mental health professionals.

In conclusion, while diet plays a crucial role in maintaining hormonal balance, it's only part of the picture. Exercise, stress management, quality sleep, awareness of environmental toxins, and nurturing social connections – they all come together to create a holistic approach to your health. Remember, it's about balance and finding what works for your unique body and lifestyle.

Chapter 7

OVERCOMING CHALLENGES

Embarking on a new dietary journey, especially one as specific as the Hormonal and Alkaline Diet for Women, is filled with potential challenges. Recognizing and preparing for these hurdles is key to your success. Let's delve into the common pitfalls and learn how to skillfully navigate them.

10 Common Pitfalls and How to Avoid Them

1. **Lack of Preparation:** Without proper meal planning, it's easy to fall back on unhealthy choices. To avoid this, spend time each week preparing a meal plan that incorporates alkaline and hormone-friendly foods.

2. **Unrealistic Expectations:** Setting unattainable goals can lead to disappointment. Be realistic about the changes you're making. Small, consistent changes often lead to long-term success.

3. **Not Understanding Your Food:** It's crucial to know which foods are alkaline-promoting and which are not. Educate yourself about food pH levels and hormonal impacts.

4. **Ignoring Body Signals:** Your body gives cues when something isn't right. Ignoring signs of hormonal imbalance can derail your efforts. Tune in to what your body is telling you.

5. **Social Eating Pressures:** Social events can challenge your

69

diet choices. Prepare by eating beforehand or bringing your hormone-friendly dishes to gatherings.

6. **Boredom with Food Choices:** Variety is the spice of life, and your diet should reflect that. Experiment with new recipes to keep your meals interesting.

7. **Neglecting Hydration:** Water is essential in maintaining pH balance. Ensure you're drinking enough water throughout the day.

8. **Overlooking the Importance of Sleep and Stress Management:** Lack of sleep and high stress can negatively impact hormonal balance. Prioritize good sleep hygiene and stress-reducing activities.

9. **Relapse into Old Eating Habits:** It's normal to slip up. Instead of seeing this as a failure, view it as a learning opportunity and get back on track.

10. **Not Seeking Support:** It's tough to do it alone. Join support groups or find a diet accountability partner.

Ways to Stay Motivated and Track Progress

1. **Set Clear, Achievable Goals:** Instead of vague objectives like "eat healthier," set specific goals like "incorporate two alkaline-rich foods into each meal."

2. **Keep a Food and Mood Journal:** Documenting your meals, how they make you feel, and any changes in your symptoms can provide insight into what works best for your body.

3. **Celebrate Small Wins:** Did you drink enough water today? Did you choose a healthy snack over a processed one? Celebrate these small victories.

4. **Visual Reminders:** Keep motivational quotes or your dietary

goals in visible places as daily reminders of your commitment.

5. **Regular Check-Ins:** Schedule weekly or monthly check-ins with yourself or a health coach to assess progress and adjust goals as needed.

6. **Educational Boost:** Continuously educate yourself about hormonal health and alkaline diets. This knowledge can be a powerful motivator.

7. **Connect with a Community:** Join online forums or local groups focused on similar dietary journeys. Sharing experiences and tips can be incredibly motivating.

8. **Track Physical Changes:** Sometimes changes are subtle. Regularly tracking your weight, energy levels, and other physical changes can highlight your progress.

9. **Embrace Flexibility:** Life is unpredictable. Being flexible with your diet while maintaining its core principles is key.

10. **Reflect on Your Journey:** Regularly reflect on why you started this journey and the benefits you've noticed since you began. This can reignite your motivation.

Remember, the journey to hormonal balance and embracing an alkaline diet is a marathon, not a sprint. Patience, persistence, and a positive mindset are your best allies in this health journey.

Chapter 8

SPECIAL CONSIDERATIONS

In this chapter, we delve into the nuanced relationship between diet, hormones, and specific life stages or conditions that women may encounter. Understanding these dynamics is crucial for tailoring the Hormonal and Alkaline Diet to meet unique needs.

Hormonal Changes Through Different Life Stages

Adolescence: This is a pivotal stage for hormonal development. A diet rich in calcium, iron, and vitamin D is crucial for growth and development. The alkaline diet, with its emphasis on fruits, vegetables, and whole grains, can provide these essential nutrients while promoting hormonal balance.

Reproductive Years: During these years, women's bodies undergo regular hormonal fluctuations. A balanced diet that stabilizes blood sugar levels is vital. Foods rich in omega-3 fatty acids, like flaxseeds and walnuts, can be beneficial. Maintaining a slightly alkaline environment in the body may help in managing premenstrual syndrome (PMS) symptoms.

Pregnancy and Breastfeeding: This period requires increased nutritional intake. The alkaline diet, with its focus on nutrient-dense foods, supports both mother and baby's health. However, it's important to consult with healthcare professionals to ensure all nutritional needs are met.

Perimenopause and Menopause: As estrogen levels fluctuate and decrease, a diet high in calcium and vitamin D becomes essential to protect bone health. Phytoestrogens found in soy products can offer some benefits. Alkaline foods can help in managing weight gain, a common issue during this stage.

Addressing Specific Conditions

Polycystic Ovary Syndrome (PCOS): Women with PCOS may benefit from a diet that regulates insulin levels, as insulin resistance is often a concern. The alkaline diet, which is low in processed foods and high in fiber, can be beneficial. Foods rich in anti-inflammatory properties, like berries and leafy greens, can also be helpful.

Menopause: During menopause, hormonal changes can lead to symptoms like hot flashes, mood swings, and weight gain. A diet rich in calcium and vitamin D is crucial for bone health. Foods that help maintain a healthy weight and balanced mood, like complex carbohydrates and omega-3 fatty acids, are also important.

Endometriosis: An alkaline diet may help manage endometriosis symptoms. Anti-inflammatory foods, such as turmeric and ginger, can be beneficial. Reducing red meat and increasing the intake of fruits, vegetables, and whole grains can also provide relief.

Thyroid Issues: Thyroid function is closely linked to diet. For those with hypothyroidism, iodine-rich foods like seaweed can be beneficial. However, it's important to avoid overconsumption. Those with hyperthyroidism might need to limit iodine intake.

Osteoporosis: A diet rich in calcium and vitamin D is essential for bone health, particularly in postmenopausal women. Alkaline foods like leafy greens and almonds can be beneficial, but it's important to balance them with adequate protein intake.

Breast Cancer: Post-diagnosis, a balanced diet plays a crucial role. Foods high in antioxidants and fiber, and low in fat, can be beneficial. Phytoestrogens have mixed reviews; it's crucial to discuss dietary changes with a healthcare provider.

In conclusion, the Hormonal and Alkaline Diet isn't a one-size-fits-all solution. Each stage of life and each condition requires a tailored approach. By understanding these nuances, women can better navigate their dietary choices to support their hormonal health through all life's stages and challenges.

Chapter 9

SUCCESS STORIES
AND TESTIMONIALS

During the compilation of this book, we carried out a survey asking women of different ages about their struggle with hormonal imbalance and their knowledge of the alkaline diet, below are what they had to tell us;

10 Real-Life Success Stories: Transformations Through Diet

1. Emily's Journey with PCOS Emily, a 28-year-old graphic designer, had been battling PCOS for years, struggling with irregular periods, weight gain, and severe acne. Desperate for a solution, she stumbled upon the concept of an alkaline diet through a friend's recommendation. Initially skeptical, she began incorporating more alkaline foods like leafy greens, nuts, and seeds while cutting out processed foods and sugars. Remarkably, within a few months, Emily noticed significant improvements. Her periods became more regular, her skin cleared up, and she lost 15 pounds. More importantly, she felt a surge in her energy levels and overall well-being. Emily's story is a testament to how dietary changes can profoundly affect hormonal disorders.

2. Sarah's Menopause Management At 51, Sarah was experiencing the full brunt of menopause. Hot flashes, night sweats, and mood swings were her daily reality. Research led her to the hormonal and alkaline diet, a path she was initially hesitant to follow. But, as she slowly replaced her regular diet with more alkaline options, she started seeing changes. Her hot flashes became less frequent, and she felt more emotionally balanced. Six months into her new diet, Sarah felt like she had regained control over her body. She became an advocate for dietary changes to manage menopause, encouraging others in her community to explore this natural approach.

3. Laura's Battle Against Fatigue Laura, a 35-year-old teacher and mother of two, was constantly tired. Blood tests revealed no specific issues, but her fatigue was relentless. After attending a seminar on hormonal health, she decided to give the alkaline diet a try. Laura meticulously planned her meals, focusing on alkaline-rich fruits, vegetables, and whole grains, while avoiding acidic foods like dairy and meat. The results were not immediate, but after several weeks, Laura started to notice a difference. She was waking up feeling more refreshed and had the energy to play with her kids after a long day at work. Laura's journey highlights the importance of diet in managing energy levels and overall health.

4. Anna's Weight Loss Journey Anna, a 42-year-old software developer, had struggled with her weight for most of her adult life. She tried various diets, but nothing seemed to work in the long term. When Anna heard about the hormonal and alkaline diet, she was intrigued but skeptical. With a history of hormonal imbalances, she wondered if this approach might be different. She began by eliminating acidic foods like pro-

cessed snacks, red meat, and sugary beverages, replacing them with alkaline foods such as quinoa, kale, and cucumbers. The first few weeks were challenging, but Anna persisted, motivated by the gradual but noticeable changes in her body. As she continued, she not only lost weight but also experienced fewer cravings and more stable energy levels throughout the day. Eight months into her new diet, Anna had lost an astonishing 30 pounds. Her journey was not just about weight loss; it was about discovering a sustainable way of eating that harmonized with her body's needs. Anna's story demonstrates the transformative power of aligning diet with hormonal health, offering hope and inspiration to others facing similar struggles.

5. Megan's Fight with Acne Megan, a 25-year-old university student, had been battling severe hormonal acne since her teens. Frustrated with conventional treatments, she explored the hormonal and alkaline diet as a last resort. Megan started by cutting out dairy and processed foods, known triggers for acne, and introduced a variety of alkaline foods like avocados, beets, and almonds. The initial weeks were tough, with little visible improvement. However, Megan remained consistent, documenting her journey and tweaking her diet as she learned more about her body's responses. Slowly, her skin started clearing up. After six months, Megan's acne had dramatically reduced, and her skin had a healthy glow. Beyond the physical transformation, Megan gained a newfound confidence and a deeper understanding of the connection between diet and skin health.

6. Rachel's Fertility Success Rachel, a 33-year-old accountant, and her husband had been trying to conceive for over two years with no success. After several consultations, Rachel

learned that her hormonal imbalances were a likely contributing factor. She was introduced to the hormonal and alkaline diet by her nutritionist. Skeptical but willing to try anything, Rachel revamped her diet, focusing on hormone-balancing foods and maintaining an alkaline environment in her body. Months passed, and while Rachel noticed improvements in her overall health, she remained cautiously hopeful about conceiving. To her joy and surprise, she became pregnant within a year of starting the diet. Rachel's story is a heartwarming example of how dietary changes can play a crucial role in fertility and overall reproductive health.

7. Beth's Mood Improvement Beth, a 47-year-old librarian, had been experiencing severe mood swings and depression. Her doctor suggested that her symptoms might be linked to hormonal imbalances. Beth decided to try the hormonal and alkaline diet, initially overwhelmed by the dietary changes but driven by a desire for a natural solution. She started incorporating more green vegetables, nuts, and seeds into her meals while reducing her intake of sugar and caffeine. Over several weeks, Beth noticed a gradual but steady improvement in her mood. She felt more emotionally stable and less prone to the sudden mood dips that had plagued her. Beth's journey illustrates how diet can be a powerful tool in managing mental health and emotional well-being.

8. Sophia's Journey with Thyroid Health Sophia, a 39-year-old graphic artist, was diagnosed with hypothyroidism. Tired of relying solely on medication, she researched alternative approaches and discovered the hormonal and alkaline diet. She gradually transitioned to a diet rich in fruits, vegetables, and whole grains, reducing her consumption of processed foods and sugars. The changes were not easy, but Sophia was deter-

mined. Within months, she began to feel more energetic, and her thyroid function tests showed significant improvement. Sophia's story is an inspiring example of how dietary choices can complement medical treatment and support thyroid health.

9. Linda's Recovery from Insomnia Linda, a 50-year-old school principal, had been struggling with insomnia for years, leaving her exhausted and irritable. After reading about the potential impact of diet on sleep, Linda decided to give the hormonal and alkaline diet a try. She started by eliminating caffeine and alcohol and introduced more magnesium-rich foods like spinach and pumpkin seeds, known for their sleep-promoting properties. The transition was challenging, especially cutting out her morning coffee, but the results were worth it. Gradually, Linda began to sleep better, waking up more refreshed and alert. Her story highlights the often-overlooked connection between diet and sleep quality.

10. Zoe's Holistic Health Transformation Zoe, a 30-year-old yoga instructor, sought a holistic approach to her persistent digestive issues and hormonal imbalances. She turned to the hormonal and alkaline diet, intrigued by its emphasis on natural, whole foods. Zoe replaced acidic foods with a plant-based, alkaline-rich diet, noticing improvements not only in her digestion but also in her overall sense of well-being. She complemented her dietary changes with regular yoga and meditation, embracing a holistic lifestyle. Zoe's transformation was not just physical; it was a journey of self-discovery and a testament to the power of integrating diet, exercise, and mindfulness for complete wellness.

We are positive these 10 true-life stories addressed some of your concerns and gave you hope as it pertains to adopting the hormonal and alkaline diet, nevertheless do note that there are more success stories in our possession but we can only showcase these few for now.

COMMON Q&A ABOUT THE HORMONAL & ALKALINE DIET

1. **Q: What is the hormonal and alkaline diet, and how does it benefit women?**

    A: This diet focuses on balancing hormones and maintaining an alkaline state in the body. It's beneficial for women as it can aid in managing hormonal imbalances, reducing inflammation, and improving overall well-being.

2. **Q: Can the alkaline diet impact menstrual health?**

    A: Absolutely. An alkaline diet can help regulate menstrual cycles and alleviate symptoms like cramps and bloating by reducing inflammation and balancing hormone levels.

3. **Q: What are the top alkaline foods recommended for hormonal balance?**

    A: Leafy greens, cucumbers, avocados, almonds, and beets are highly recommended for their alkalizing properties and nutrient content.

4. **Q: How does diet influence hormonal acne?**

    A: Diet plays a crucial role. Foods high in sugar and dairy can trigger hormonal fluctuations leading to acne. An alkaline diet helps stabilize these hormones.

5. **Q: Is soy beneficial or harmful for hormonal health?**

    A: Soy contains phytoestrogens, which can mimic estrogen. It can be beneficial in moderation, but it's important to consult with a healthcare provider, especially for those with estrogen-sensitive conditions.

6. **Q: Can this diet aid in weight management?**

    A: Yes, by promoting a healthy metabolism and reducing cravings for unhealthy foods, this diet can be a powerful tool for weight management.

7. **Q: Are there any risks associated with an alkaline diet?**

    A: If not balanced properly, it might lead to a lack of essential nutrients. It's important to ensure a varied and balanced diet.

8. **Q: How quickly can one see results from following this diet?**

    A: Results vary, but many report feeling more energetic and balanced within a few weeks.

9. **Q: What's the role of hydration in the alkaline diet?**

    A: Hydration is key. It aids in maintaining an alkaline state and supports overall hormonal balance.

10. **Q: Can an alkaline diet improve fertility?**

    A: It can, by balancing hormones and creating a healthier overall body environment, which is conducive to fertility.

11. Q: How does stress affect hormonal balance and how can diet help?

A: Stress can disrupt hormonal equilibrium. A balanced diet rich in magnesium and B vitamins can help manage stress levels.

12. Q: Are there specific foods to avoid for hormonal health?

A: Yes, reducing the intake of processed foods, sugars, and high-glycemic-index foods is advisable.

13. Q: Can this diet help with menopause symptoms?

A: Definitely. It can alleviate symptoms like hot flashes and mood swings by stabilizing hormones.

14. Q: What supplements are recommended alongside this diet?

A: Vitamin D, Omega-3 fatty acids, and probiotics are often recommended, but it's best to consult with a healthcare professional.

15. Q: How does an alkaline diet affect gut health?

A: It promotes a healthy gut by encouraging the growth of beneficial bacteria, which is essential for hormonal balance.

16. Q: Can this diet impact sleep quality?

A: Yes, by promoting hormonal balance and reducing stress, it can improve sleep quality.

17. Q: How important is organic food in this diet?

A: Organic foods are less likely to contain hormone-disrupting pesticides, making them a better choice for this diet.

18. Q: What are some easy ways to start transitioning to this diet?

A: Start by gradually incorporating more alkaline foods into your diet and reducing acidic foods like meats and dairy.

19. Q: Can exercise complement this diet for hormonal health?

A: Absolutely. Regular exercise can enhance the diet's effects on hormonal balance.

20. Q: How can one monitor the success of this diet?

A: Monitoring energy levels, menstrual cycle regularity, and over-all well-being can be effective indicators.

21. Q: How does this diet impact insulin sensitivity?

A: It can improve insulin sensitivity by stabilizing blood sugar levels, which is crucial for hormonal balance.

22. Q: Are there specific foods that help with thyroid health?

A: Foods rich in iodine, selenium, and zinc, like seaweed, Brazil nuts, and pumpkin seeds, are beneficial for thyroid health.

23. Q: How can this diet address PMS symptoms?

A: By balancing hormones and reducing inflammation, this diet can alleviate PMS symptoms like mood swings and bloating.

24. Q: Can the alkaline diet help with hair and skin health?

A: Yes, the diet's focus on nutrient-rich foods can improve hair and skin health by nourishing the body from within.

25. Q: What role do antioxidants play in this diet?

A: Antioxidants combat oxidative stress, which can disrupt hormonal balance. They're vital in this diet.

26. Q: How does this diet cater to postmenopausal women?

A: It helps manage postmenopausal symptoms by maintaining hormonal balance and bone health.

27. Q: What are the benefits of fermented foods in this diet?

A: Fermented foods enhance gut health, which is directly linked to hormonal balance.

28. Q: How does the alkaline diet impact mental health?

A: A balanced diet can improve mental health by stabilizing mood-regulating hormones like serotonin and dopamine.

29. Q: Are there natural sweeteners recommended in this diet?

A: Natural sweeteners like stevia and honey are preferred over refined sugars.

30. Q: How does this diet support adrenal health?

A: It reduces adrenal fatigue by balancing stress hormones and providing essential nutrients.

31. Q: Can this diet reduce the risk of hormonal cancers?

A: While no diet can guarantee cancer prevention, maintaining hormonal balance can reduce certain risk factors.

32. Q: What is the role of fiber in the hormonal and alkaline diet?

A: Fiber aids in digestion and the elimination of toxins, which is essential for hormonal balance.

33. Q: How important is portion control in this diet?

A: Portion control helps maintain a healthy weight, crucial for hormonal equilibrium.

34. Q: Can this diet aid in recovery post-pregnancy?

A: Yes, it can support hormonal rebalancing and provide vital nutrients for postpartum recovery.

35. Q: What impact does this diet have on bone health?

A: Alkaline diets rich in calcium and magnesium can promote bone health and prevent osteoporosis.

36. Q: How does the diet help in managing PCOS?

A: It helps in managing PCOS by stabilizing insulin and androgen levels.

37. Q: Are there any quick alkaline snacks recommended?

A: Almonds, carrot sticks, and hummus are great alkaline snack options.

38. Q: How can one ensure protein intake in this diet?

A: Include plant-based proteins like lentils, quinoa, and tofu for adequate protein intake.

39. Q: What is the importance of omega-3 fatty acids in this diet?

A: Omega-3s reduce inflammation and support hormonal health, especially for brain and heart function.

40. Q: Can this diet improve energy levels throughout the day?

A: Yes, stabilizing blood sugar levels, can lead to sustained energy throughout the day.

41. Q: How does the alkaline diet affect cholesterol levels?

A: It can help lower bad cholesterol levels by promoting a healthy diet and lifestyle.

42. Q: Are there specific meal timing strategies recommended?

A: Eating at regular intervals can help maintain blood sugar and hormone levels.

43. Q: How can this diet be customized for athletes?

A: Athletes may need more protein and carbohydrates, which can be adjusted within the diet's framework.

44. Q: What are the best hydration practices in this diet?

A: Drinking alkaline water and herbal teas can support hydration needs.

45. Q: How does this diet interact with common medications?

A: It's generally safe, but always consult with a doctor, especially if on medication for hormonal imbalances.

46. Q: Can the alkaline diet aid in detoxification?

A: Yes, it supports the body's natural detoxification processes by providing antioxidants and aiding liver function.

47. Q: How should one handle dining out while following this diet?

A: Choose dishes rich in vegetables and lean proteins, and avoid processed or sugary foods.

48. Q: Are there specific spices or herbs that enhance this diet?

A: Herbs like turmeric and ginger are beneficial for their anti-inflammatory properties.

49. Q: How can one transition back to a regular diet after achieving hormonal balance?

A: Transition gradually while maintaining key principles like eating whole foods and managing portion sizes.

50. Q: What advice do you have for maintaining this diet long-term?

A: Focus on variety and balance, listen to your body, and make adjustments as needed for sustainable health.

CONCLUSION

As we conclude our journey through understanding the hormonal and alkaline diet for women, it's important to reflect on the key takeaways and look forward to maintaining a healthy hormonal balance through diet and lifestyle.

Summarizing Key Takeaways

1. Understanding the Hormone-Diet Connection: We've explored how hormones, those powerful chemical messengers in our body, are significantly influenced by what we eat. A diet rich in alkaline foods helps to maintain the pH balance of the body, which is crucial for optimal hormonal function.

2. The Essentials of an Alkaline Diet: We delved into the principles of the alkaline diet, emphasizing foods that are high in minerals and low in acid-forming compounds. This includes a bounty of fruits, vegetables, nuts, and seeds.

3. Impact of Diet on Hormonal Health: It's clear that our dietary choices have a profound impact on our hormonal health. Foods like leafy greens, cruciferous vegetables, and healthy fats are beneficial, while processed foods, excessive sugar, and caffeine can be disruptive.

4. Holistic Approach to Health: Beyond diet, we emphasized the importance of a holistic approach – incorporating exercise, stress management, and adequate sleep, all of which play a pivotal role in hormonal balance.

5. Individualized Approach: We acknowledged the uniqueness of each individual. What works for one woman may not work for another. It's important to listen to your body and possibly consult with a healthcare provider to tailor the diet to your specific needs.

The Journey Ahead: Maintaining Hormonal Health

As you continue on your journey towards maintaining hormonal health, remember that this is a continuous process, not a one-time fix. Here are some strategies to keep in mind:

1. Consistency is Key: Integrating the principles of an alkaline diet into your daily routine is more beneficial than sporadic healthy eating. Consistency leads to lasting change.

2. Stay Informed and Adaptable: New research in nutrition and hormonal health is constantly emerging. Stay informed and be open to adjusting your diet and lifestyle as new information becomes available.

3. Mindful Eating: Pay attention to how your body reacts to certain foods. Mindful eating helps in recognizing foods that positively or negatively affect your hormonal balance.

4. Support System: Surround yourself with a supportive community, whether it's friends, family, or online groups. Sharing experiences and tips can be incredibly motivating.

5. Regular Health Check-Ups: Regular consultations with healthcare professionals can help in monitoring your hormonal health and making necessary adjustments in your diet and lifestyle.

6. Embrace the Journey: Remember, this journey is as much about mental and emotional well-being as it is about physical

health. Embrace the process and be kind to yourself along the way.

In closing, the hormonal and alkaline diet is not just about what you eat; it's about creating a balanced lifestyle that nurtures your body, mind, and spirit. As you continue to apply these principles, you're not just enhancing your hormonal health; you're embarking on a path to a more vibrant, healthy, and fulfilling life.

APPENDIX

A. Additional Resources

1. Nutritional Websites and Blogs

    *   NutritionFacts.org: Evidence-based nutritional information.

    *   The Hormone Health Network: Comprehensive hormone health resources.

2. Online Communities and Forums

    *   Women's Health Forums: A platform for discussing women's health and diet.

    *   Reddit: Subreddits like r/Nutrition and r/Hormones for community advice.

3. Mobile Apps

    *   MyFitnessPal: For tracking diet and nutritional intake.

    *   Hormone Horoscope: An app providing daily insights into how hormones affect the body.

4. Books and Publications

    *   "The Complete Hormone Puzzle Cookbook" by Kela Smith

    *   "The pH Miracle: Balance Your Diet, Reclaim Your Health" by Robert O. Young

5. References

    *   O'Neill, Barbara. "Self Heal by Design."

- Brown, Susan E. "The Acid Alkaline Food Guide." Square One Publishers, 2013.

- Northrup, Christiane. "Women's Bodies, Women's Wisdom: Creating Physical and Emotional Health and Healing." Bantam, 2010.

- Romm, Aviva. "The Adrenal Thyroid Revolution: A Proven 4-Week Program to Rescue Your Metabolism, Hormones, Mind & Mood." HarperOne, 2017.

- Turner, Natasha. "The Hormone Diet: A 3-Step Program to Help You Lose Weight, Gain Strength, and Live Younger Longer." Rodale Books, 2011.

- Vitti, Alisa. "WomanCode: Perfect Your Cycle, Amplify Your Fertility, Supercharge Your Sex Drive, and Become a Power Source." HarperOne, 2013.

- Lee, John R., and Virginia Hopkins. "What Your Doctor May Not Tell You About Menopause: The Breakthrough Book on Natural Hormone Balance." Warner Books, 2004.

- Hechtman, Leah. "Clinical Naturopathic Medicine." Churchill Livingstone, 2012.

- Briden, Lara. "Period Repair Manual: Natural Treatment for Better Hormones and Better Periods." Greenpeak Publishing, 2017.

- Young, Robert O., and Shelley Redford Young. "The pH Miracle for Weight Loss: Balance Your Body Chemistry, Achieve Your Ideal Weight." Grand Central Publishing, 2006.

- Gates, Donna, and Linda Schatz. "The Body Ecology Diet: Recovering Your Health and Rebuilding Your Immunity." Hay House, 2011.

B - avacado toast / bread / egg

L - chicken + veg soup   bread
                          or quinoa

D - protein
         asp.
      sweet potato

Snack fruit
       almonds
      dark choc.

Nick pivoted. Leaning his elbow on the rail, he tried to remain casual as he looked at Kate and listened to her proposition. Acting only mildly interested, he asked, "This beach, does it have waves?"

"Oh, yeah," Kate nodded, her eyes brightening. "Much bigger waves than the Gulf."

"I'm listening," Nick said, his body inching closer to Kate's.

"You can watch the storms roll in," Kate added.

"Sunsets?" Nick pressed.

"Oh sure, *and* sunrise," Kate smiled.

"Sunrise, all right," Nick nodded. "I like sunrises, too."

"You'll have to travel, but we can arrange free room and board," Kate said.

"Free room and board?" Nick exclaimed with a grin. "You know, that is the holy grail for a vagabond surfer."

"Oh, you're no vagabond, Nick Mason," Kate smiled into his eyes.